the living + active challenge

YOUR 5-WEEK TRAINING GUIDE FOR BODY AND SOUL

Contents

WELCOME

What's up, everyone?! I am so glad you've chosen to take your fitness another step deeper by purchasing this "Living and Active" experience training guide! While the free resources on my blog (www.claresmith.me) are super helpful, I feel like this will take your efforts an extra mile!

This training guide is a place meant for you to write down what you are going through, track progress, and keep you on track. It's easy to start a plan, but keeping it up can be so hard! This training guide will be a huge part in your success over the next five weeks. (Plus, there are two BONUS workouts at the end!)

If you have a bad week, that's OK! That is to be expected during a 5-week challenge like this one. You can choose to pick up where you left off, or start over again. Check out the "bonus" section below for where to print off blank copies of the calendar!

In case you don't know (or need reminded!) the focus of this specific challenge is to be consistent in two areas for five weeks: scripture memorization and exercise. (I don't hit eating on this challenge but feel free to add a new goal for you in that area!)

This challenge is done live on my blog one time a year. If you are doing it live, then you are eligible for the grand prize packages! If you are doing this on your own, consider teaming up with friends at church or work and create your own prize package and check-in system!

For those of you doing the challenge live on my blog, in order to qualify for the GRAND PRIZE, you must do two things: memorize the weekly scripture and exercise four times a week for a minimum of 25 minutes. Then check-in weekly (on the blog!) to let me know that you did those two things! At the end of the five weeks, those who have successfully memorized scripture and exercised (and checked in!) will be eligible to win! If you want to print off the verses, check out my blog where you can do so!

The training guide is divided up weekly so that you can "win small!" Five weeks is a long time to stay committed and motivated which is why I want you to take it week by week.

READ IT: Read your weekly verses (you only need to memorize one) and the devotional with it.
DO IT: Write out your week's plan and then refer to it daily!
LIVE IT: This is your chance to journal as you go through the challenge.
WORK IT: A tip or recipe to help you "sharpen" your health and work it out!

Let's start this challenge off with a prayer! Reference this often when you are upset, challenged, or feeling good! We must stay connected to the source of life and freedom in order to transfer that to our physical health!

Heavenly Father, thank you so much for this challenge. Thank you for what you are going to teach me during these five weeks. I know that you have equipped me for this journey through your Word and the support of those around me. Help me to lean on You every day and to renew my mind every morning as I learn new techniques and insights about myself! You created my life and knew this challenge would be a part of it even during my time in mama's womb. Thank you for your sovereignty and carrying me through all the way. To your glory and for your kingdom, may my health be a sacrifice unto you. Amen

TRAIN HARD. EAT WELL. LIVE FREE!

Clare

p.s. Redeem social media during these five weeks to aid you in your health instead of deter it! Follow me on Facebook (@claresmithofficial), instagram (@claresmithofficial), twitter (@claresmith__), pinterest (@claresmith_) , youtube (@claresmithofficial), and periscope (@claresmith)! I would love to hear from you so use the hashtag #livingandactive so I can see how you're doing!

BONUS: I have a special page on my blog for those of you who purchased this book! You can watch a video of how each of the exercises should be completed and a printable document of BLANK calendars so you can personalize this challenge as many times as you want! Go to: http://www.claresmith.me/livingandactiveresources/ password: ilovefreestuff (all lowercase and no blanks!)

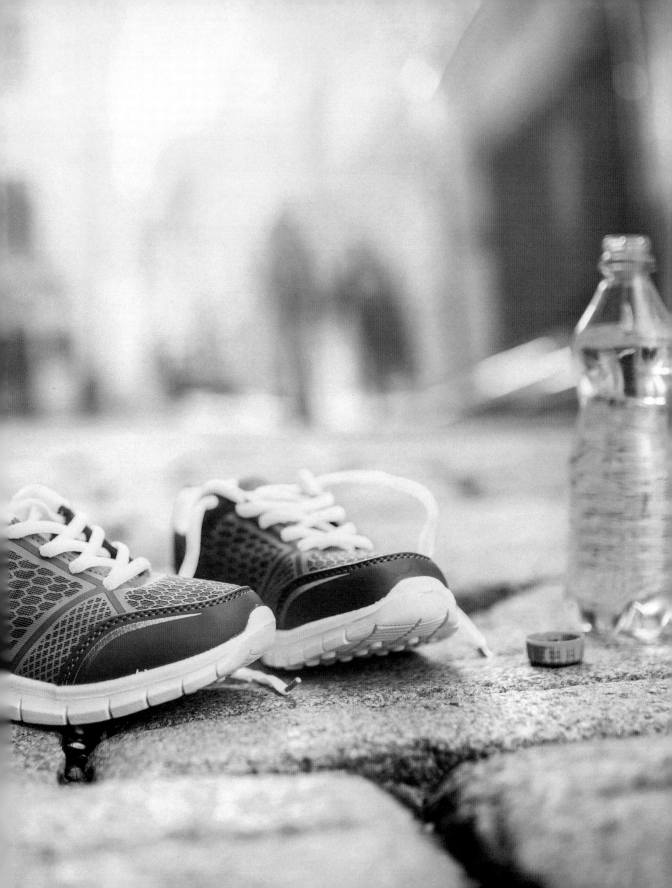

LET'S GET STARTED

---

1 | Print off a copy of the full month blank calendar so that you can personalize it and make it real! (Check out the "bonus" section in the welcome portion of this guide for how to access it!)

2 | Take measurements! The measurements section below is so important! I know you won't want to do them at the beginning of the challenge, but it will be a nice tool at the end! (Check out the definitions and sample page at the end if you aren't sure how to take measurements!)

3 | Find an accountability partner (or a few!) Write their name(s) here.

_____   _____   _____

4 | Figure out your workout routine for week 1 and write it in week 1's calendar! Reference my website for some routines, check out the bonus workouts at the end, or continue with your own plan!

MEASUREMENTS

WEEK 1: DATE _____   WEEK 5: DATE _____

CHEST: _____   CHEST: _____
WAIST: _____   WAIST: _____
HIPS: _____   HIPS: _____
THIGHS: _____   THIGHS: _____
WEIGHT: _____   WEIGHT: _____

WEEK ONE

Tied Together

"Though one may be overpowered, two can defend themselves.
A cord of three strands is not quickly broken."

ECCLESIASTES 4:12

"As iron sharpens iron so one person sharpens another."

PROVERBS 27:17

READ IT.

When I was praying through which key points that I wanted to take us through for this 5 week challenge, I knew that this would be the first week. I know the importance of being "Tied Together" in both my physical and spiritual life. We cannot do this journey alone. God has not created us for that! We are to have some solid folks whom we can trust that to keep us strong.

My best friend, college roommate and running partner, Leslie, keeps me going. I am not much of a distance runner (Sure, I've done a few half-marathons, but it's not really my thing!) and I would quit (or not go) if it weren't for the fact that she was running with me. I also have a few other friends who are very active and knowing that we all enjoy living a life of physical fitness, really does encourage me in the journey.
I also have this in my spiritual life, as I'm part of a "Good Morning Girls" group. We check-in every morning with what we are reading in our Bibles. Left to my own, I would not keep on top of it. I would drift and the next thing you know, I'm a week or two off from getting in God's Word.

It's the nature of the beast.

In the verse that I have us memorizing, it talks about a 3-stranded cord. What a wonderful visual reminder for us.

WE ARE STRONGER TOGETHER THAN WE ARE APART.

The cords are not strong laying beside each other. They aren't strong while laying on top of one another or being end to end. The strength is in the weaving and intertwining of the three.

I know that it can be hard to get that close especially if you've been burned in the past, but God is faithful and will provide the right people at the right time! And let's not forget the most important strand of this cord--God. Without Him, you will fail miserably! That's why this challenge is more than just the physical, but is also a challenge for our spiritual lives. I want us to incorporate and weave BOTH areas together!

Many of you have someone who you are "Tied Together" with for this challenge and that's wonderful. But for those of you who don't, take a minute now and ask God to bring someone in your path.

DO IT.

DAY	SUN	MON	TUE	WED	THUR	FRI	SAT
WORKOUT *include what you did, when you'll do it, and how long it lasts* am/pm ___ min	am/pm ___ min	am/pm ___ min	am/pm ___ min	am/pm ___ min	am/pm ___ min	am/pm ___ min	am/pm ___ min
SCRIPTURE PRACTICE	☐	☐	☐	☐	☐	☐	☐

Challenge: Find at least one other person to join you on the "Living and Active" challenge. Commit to checking in with each other twice a week in both areas (physically and spiritually)

Journal: _____

_____

_____

_____

_____

_____

_____

_____

_____

_____

_____

Non-Scale Victories:

How often should I workout and what should I do? Use this acronym, GIDDY, and ask these questions, then GIDDY up to it!

G: GOALS: What are they?

Do you want to lose fat? Gain muscle? Increase endurance? Work on flexibility? Have fun? Connect with someone?

I: INTERESTS: What do you like?

Dancing? Lifting? Running? Hiking? Outside? Inside? Pilates?

D: DAYS: What days a week can you commit to 90% of the time?

Don't overshoot this. Be realistic

D: DURATION: How long can you workout at a time?

15 minutes 2 times a day? 30 minutes a day? 60 minutes?

Y: YOU: How do YOU feel about this workout?

Does this fill your cup? Challenge you? Bring you closer to your family? Keep you from sin?

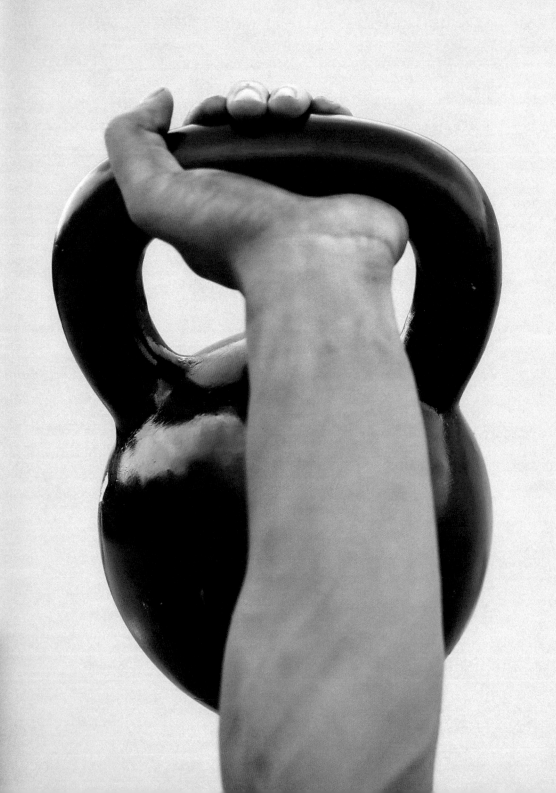

WEEK TWO

Dedicated Daily

"Therefore do not worry about tomorrow, for tomorrow will worry about itself.
Each day has enough trouble of its own."

MATTHEW 6:34

"Because of the Lord's great love we are not consumed, for his compassions
never fail. They are new every morning; great is your faithfulness."

LAMENTATIONS 3:22-23

READ IT.

Lifetime consistency is one of the biggest roadblocks I see with those in their health journeys. Once someone is derailed--even if it's for a day or two--it's so easy to give up. I see this time and time again and what happens is instead of getting back on the wagon, they get off and stay off. It's a vicious cycle that is so defeating.

Here's what I've found. **WE TRY TO STORE UP STRENGTH IN BATCHES**. We think that if we work really hard for three days, that it will buy us another three in focus and willpower. We do this in our spiritual lives too. I can think of times when I've been very consistent daily in asking God for strength and wisdom in a particular situation or with someone God has placed in my life. Then once the urgency leaves, I stop asking, relying on the past week's prayers to get me through.

There's nothing in the Christian walk that talks about storing up anything. We can't store up grace for the day. We can't store up strength. We can't store up anything. **EVERYTHING IS A DAILY COMMITMENT.** We take up our cross daily (Luke 9:23). We ask for our daily bread (not weekly!) (Matthew 6:11) There's a great story in Exodus that helped give me that "aha" moment that I needed.

Moses and the Israelites were in the desert. The Lord provided manna and gave specific instructions to Moses. "Each one is to gather as much as he needs..." (v.16), but that "No one was to keep any of it until morning" (v.19). For those who disregarded the instructions and kept the manna until morning, theirs rotted and began to smell. (READ Exodus 16 for more.)

2 IMPORTANT THINGS HERE:

1 | They had to go out an of their tents to gather it. It didn't come FedEx to the tent door. Their friend or husband didn't give it to them. It was their job to go out.

2 | They gathered what they needed for THAT DAY. Nothing more. Nothing less. They did not store up for tomorrow.

We have a great responsibility to ask God for the strength, grace and wisdom for the day. Then we need to take what He gives us for that day. Nothing more. Nothing less. We can't rely upon others to give us what we need to be getting for ourselves either.

The best advice I can give you is this: Wake up. Pray immediately for strength and wisdom. Do your best during the day. Go to bed, thanking Him for what He gave you. Wake up. Repeat.

Daily. Daily. Daily.

DO IT.

DAY	SUN	MON	TUE	WED	THUR	FRI	SAT
WORKOUT *include what you did, when you'll do it, and how long it lasts*	am/pm ___ min	am/pm ___ min	am/pm ___ min	am/pm ___ min	am/pm ___ min	am/pm ___ min	am/pm ___ min
SCRIPTURE PRACTICE	☐	☐	☐	☐	☐	☐	☐

LIVE IT.

Challenge: Bookend your day in prayer for strength and wisdom for the day. Before bed, do a little mental review of how you did that day in your marriage, health, parenting etc so that it helps you as you focus the next day.

Journal: _____

_____

_____

_____

_____

_____

_____

_____

_____

_____

_____

_____

_____

Non-Scale Victories:

WORK IT.

Meal Prep for Success! I keep a few things in my fridge and freezer to ensure healthy eating! I make up a lot of frozen turkey burgers, a veggie tray, hard-boiled eggs, portioned out sizes of nuts, and a big salad every week! You'll find that it's much easier to eat healthy foods when you have them at your finger-tips so take the time out every week to prep and meal plan! If that sounds exhausting, just pick ONE of those things and do it consistently for the rest of the challenge!

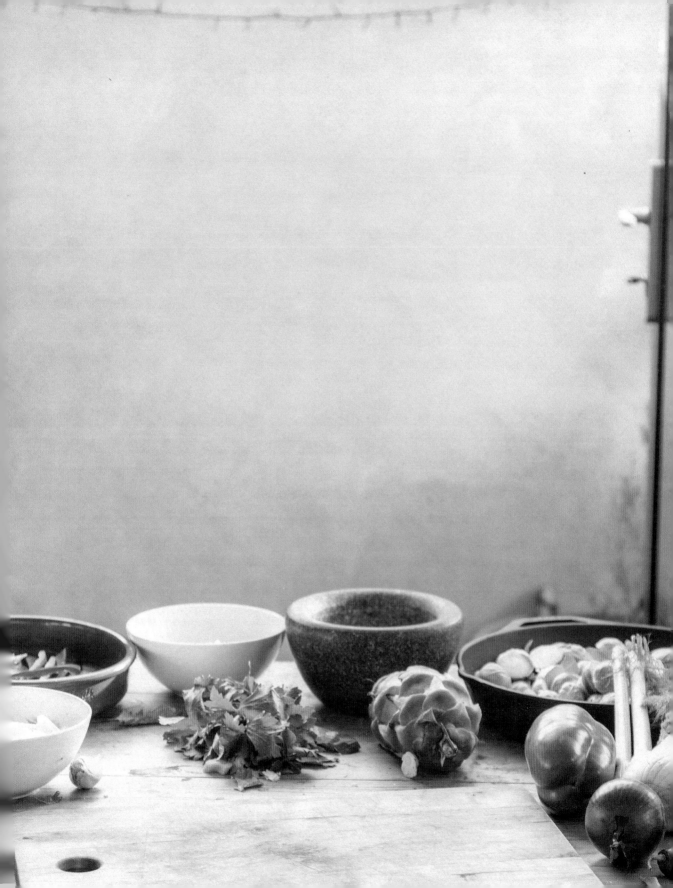

WEEK THREE

Craving Conquerors

"For everything in the world- the cravings of sinful man, the lust of his eyes and the boasting of what he has and does-comes not from the Father but from the world."

1 JOHN 2:16

"For he satisfies the longing soul, and the hungry soul he fills with good things."

PSALM 107:9

READ IT.

Craving: an intense desire or longing

I bet you've had one, or a HUNDRED in your lifetime! I know that I have! And boy, those cravings can get us into trouble, can't they?

We want to conquer cravings because we don't want anything controlling or conquering us! I could write many posts on cravings (and I plan on giving more info through this week), but I want to start this week out with a few thoughts.

1 | ALL CRAVINGS AREN'T BAD. BAD CRAVINGS ARE BAD.

There are times when I would tell you to give into your craving. Maybe it's a need for a rich, deep piece of chocolate after a wonderful dinner, or a lightly seasoned avocado alongside some lean steak. (Yes, I crave these things!) Or, maybe, the craving is for those in your life to taste and see the beauty of Christ's love. 1 Peter 2:2 even tells us to CRAVE pure spiritual milk. We need to be prayerful about our cravings and check them against God's standards. (1 John 2:16 tells us that the cravings of SINFUL man come from the world.)

2 | MANY TIMES CRAVINGS ARE A SIGN THAT SOMETHING ELSE IS LACKING.

Cravings in our life, be it physical, emotional, or relational, are often a reflection of something lacking in our lives. I plan on sharing some scientific stuff with you this week about cravings, but what you'll find is that we are missing something in another area of life. By satisfying the RIGHT craving, we can put to bed the wrong one. When we crave attention from our friends, we often are lacking in self-esteem. When we crave many sweets, we are often lacking from (the right) type of carbs. The list could go on. We need to identify those times when we have cravings to see if they match up with another area we are lacking in.

3 | CRAVINGS WILL PASS.

Oh, they may not seem like they will, but they will pass. 1 John 2:17 tells us that the world and its desires pass away. We need to stand strong, understanding that cravings are usually a temporary fix. If we can get through the rough spot (by leaving, changing our focus, or praying) then we will be victorious!

DO IT.

DAY	SUN	MON	TUE	WED	THUR	FRI	SAT
WORKOUT *include what you did, when you'll do it, and how long it lasts*	*am/pm* ___ *min*	*am/pm* ___ *min*	*am/pm* ___ *min*	*am/pm* ___ *min*	*am/pm* ___ *min*	*am/pm* ___ *min*	*am/pm* ___ *min*
SCRIPTURE PRACTICE	☐	☐	☐	☐	☐	☐	☐

WEEK THREE

Challenge: List your top three cravings (not just food oriented!). List when you have them (after dinner, after seeing a friend, after work etc). Are these cravings from the world? Are they coming from a sin nature? If yes, then commit to praying about them. Consider talking with a close friend about them. Manage and control your cravings! Don't ever let them take control of you!

Journal: _____

_____

_____

_____

_____

_____

_____

_____

_____

_____

_____

Non-Scale Victories:

Did you know? Cocoa is proven to help conquer cravings! It raises the levels of dopamine and serotonin, which relaxes the body and changes the brain chemistry! Add 1-2 tablespoons to your protein shake or make your own "hot cocoa!" Take 1-2 tablespoons, pour hot water slowly into it, stir in your favorite sweetener, cinnamon or even cayenne pepper and sip away!

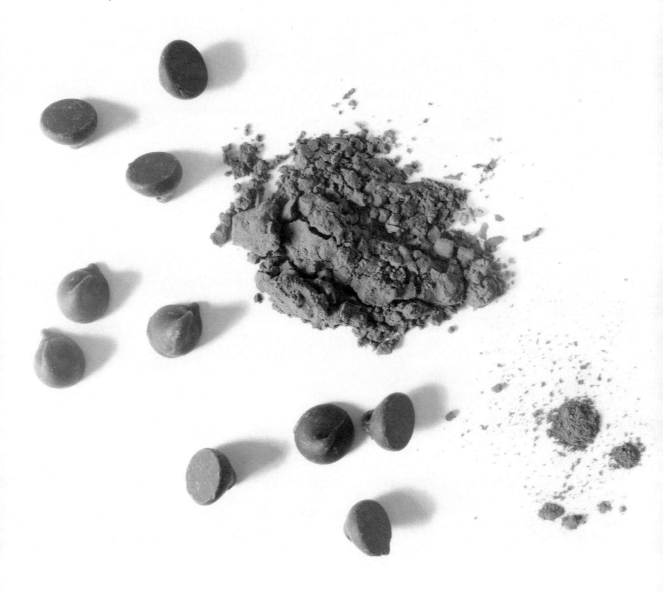

WEEK FOUR

Heart Healthy

"Above all else, guard your heart for it is the wellspring of life."

PROVERBS 4:23

"My flesh and my heart may fail, but God is the strength of my heart and my portion forever."

PSALM 73:26

READ IT.

I'm sure you aren't surprised that a fitness challenge has something to do with the heart. And while our physical hearts need to be healthy, so does our spiritual hearts. Many people don't relate the two as a source of issues with their physical lives, but after dealing with years and years of women and their weight loss challenges, I'm here to tell you that they are in fact related.

Our soul food this week tells us that the heart is the WELLSPRING of life! The WELLSPRING! It is from the heart that everything comes forth and so if we have a sickness in it, then why are we surprised that the infection has spread throughout the rest of the body?

Each of us have our own set of heart issues to deal with. They look different for each person, so the route in which you take to fix them will look different, too.

Having a heart that is not well will affect us in many areas. Let me throw a few questions out to you. See if you can relate:

- Are you holding onto some harsh words that someone in your past has said about your body?
- Are you trying to keep up with your friends around you either in career, status, or looks?
- Has your marriage taken a turn for the worse, causing you to retreat to an unhealthy lifestyle?
- Are worries about your future keeping you from living life to the fullest now?

Worry, comparison, discontent, a misguided self-image....these things all take our heart and make them unhealthy. And in return, that spills out into our physical life. Many of us turn to food, or retreat, (causing us to be inactive) and so goes the vicious cycle.

We need to get down and dirty. Band-aids don't work. Surgery does. It takes a skilled team to help you through it, and it takes time.

Take this challenge to heart (no pun intended!), and after you get through it, then consider talking with someone who is trained to help you. At a minimum, find a friend who can walk through these hurts with you and help you find that healthy heart that you need. .

DO IT.

DAY	SUN	MON	TUE	WED	THUR	FRI	SAT
WORKOUT *include what you did, when you'll do it, and how long it lasts* am/pm ___ min	am/pm ___ min	am/pm ___ min	am/pm ___ min	am/pm ___ min	am/pm ___ min	am/pm ___ min	
SCRIPTURE PRACTICE	☐	☐	☐	☐	☐	☐	☐

Challenge: It's time for some self-inventory. I want you to pray and then write a response to this sometime this week. Don't expect all the answers to come to you right now. The Holy Spirit will work and guide you.

Past: Are there hurts, pains or words that repeat over in your mind? Think back to your younger years...ages 8, 13, 17, etc; Current: What current habits do you have now that are a reaction to your worries and hurts? Eating when sad? Retreating when hurt? Lashing out when angry? Future: What future worries are you carrying that cause you to not live in the moment? Where do you have anxiety and unrest?

Journal: _____

_____

_____

_____

_____

_____

_____

_____

_____

_____

Non-Scale Victories:

The crockpot is a busy woman's best friend! I use it all the time and it really ensures that we have a healthy meal waiting for us when we get home from a busy day. It's also super helpful if you want to make a lot of food and freeze it. Soups are perfect to freeze in individual (or larger!) portions and pull out on a day when you don't feel like cooking for lunch or dinner! Here is a very basic crockpot recipe I use all the time!

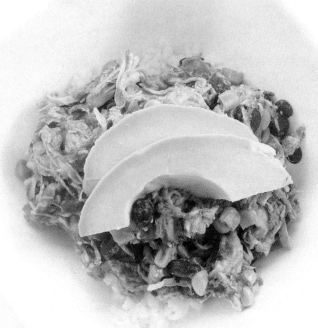

MEXI-CHICKEN

1-2 lbs of chicken breast

1 can of black beans (drained)

1 can of corn (drained) or 1/2 frozen bag

1 jar of salsa (or use 1 can of diced tomatoes)

salt, pepper, and any other seasonings you may like (such as taco!)

Add all of it in a crockpot and cook on low for 6-8 hours. Shred the chicken with 2 forks before you serve and mix it all together. Serve over rice, in a tortilla, or make a salad with it! Garnish with cilantro, shredded cheese, greek yogurt (or cream cheese if you want to go crazy!)

WEEK FIVE

Marathon Minded

"May God himself, the God of peace, sanctify you through and through. May your whole spirit, soul and body be kept blameless at the coming of our Lord Jesus Christ"

1 THESSALONIANS 5:23

"Let us not become weary in doing good, for at the proper time we will reap a harvest if we do not give up."

GALATIANS 6:9

READ IT.

Are you ready to sign up for 26.2 miles? KIDDING! I'm not going to make you run a marathon...at least physically. But I am going to encourage you to run one emotionally and spiritually!

I wish I could count the number of folks I see who each have quit in their health journey. I have seen disappointment and defeat written all over their faces. The focus is short term, therefore the commitment is short lived.

We have many, many years over the course of our lives to change, improve, mature, and achieve. Yet, we find ourselves in these short sprints with lots of intensity and major burnout.

Our society doesn't do a good job of helping us out either. We live among a "want it, get it" mentality. Most things we want are at the touch of our fingers. You want that app? Buy it now. You want a book? Download it immediately for your Kindle. You want to lose weight? Take this pill for seven days.

We are no longer trained to think long term in life. We have lost the art of becoming marathon minded! But as Believers in Christ, we are to be transformed in our thinking! We are all running a race--and it's a race that keeps going until we reach Him!

How we do we stay marathon-minded? By being daily dedicated! The irony in it all is that to keep going long-term, we have to reset short-term! Find what works for your life and current phase of life. Find exercise you enjoy that involves people you want to be around. Ask God to give you a marathon perspective while living a day-to-day life.

I encourage you to stay in the race. Whether it's your marriage, children, health, or spiritual issues. Are you with me?

DO IT.

DAY	SUN	MON	TUE	WED	THUR	FRI	SAT
WORKOUT *include what you did, when you'll do it, and how long it lasts*	am/pm ___ min	am/pm ___ min	am/pm ___ min	am/pm ___ min	am/pm ___ min	am/pm ___ min	am/pm ___ min
SCRIPTURE PRACTICE	☐	☐	☐	☐	☐	☐	☐

Challenge: Is there an area of life that you have justified "quitting" in? Maybe you haven't intentionally quit, but you've stopped praying and putting intention in it. Take a second to think through some of these areas. Ask God for endurance until He comes!

Ex: Marriage, children, health, salvation/spiritual health of loved ones

Journal: _____

_____

_____

_____

_____

_____

_____

_____

_____

_____

Non-Scale Victories:

Rev up your playlist! Music is key to most people's workouts. In fact, if you just add one song to your workout playlist, you can burn an additional 50-60 calories if you keep going! I find that I have to keep mine switched up about every month or so so if you have found yourself bored during your workouts, then make this small switch! My favorites are TobyMac, Lecrae, Andy Mineo, and Hillsong Young & Free and I love going "old-school" with songs that I listened to 4 or even 15 years ago!

Here is a quick 26 minute playlist for you to try!

HEAVEN BY GROUP 1 CREW   **STOMP** BY KIRK FRANKLIN

VIP BY MANIC DRIVE   **IGNITION** BY TOBYMAC

THE SAINTS BY ANDY MINEO   **WAKE** BY HILLSONG YOUNG & FREE

SAMPLES +
DEFINITIONS

Here is a look at how your weekly glance might look like!

DAY	SUN	MON	TUE	WED	THUR	FRI	SAT
WORKOUT *include what you did, when you'll do it, and how long it lasts*	full body strength training	pilates & sprints	full body strength training	pilates & elliptical	OFF	long run	OFF
	(am)/pm	(am)/pm	(am)/pm	(am)/pm	am/pm	(am)/pm	am/pm
	60 min	40 min	50 min	40 min	0 min	45 min	0 min
SCRIPTURE PRACTICE	☑	☑	☐	☑	☐	☑	☑

DEFINITIONS:

NON-SCALE VICTORIES (NSV): These are exactly as they say…victories in your health which don't include a scale! Some examples might be clothing fitting looser, eating one scoop of ice cream instead of two, consistent weekly workouts etc. Don't forget about mindset NSV's too! Getting right back on track if you have a bad day, talking yourself through that rough workout, and thinking differently about your body!

HOW TO MEASURE YOUR BODY:

CHEST: Measure directly under your breasts, as high up as possible.

WAIST: Measure at its narrowest point width-wise, usually just above the navel.

HIPS: Measure around the widest part of the hipbones.

THIGHS: Measure around fullest part of upper leg while standing

WEIGHT: Step on a scale and record weight. If you can get body fat tested, do that too!

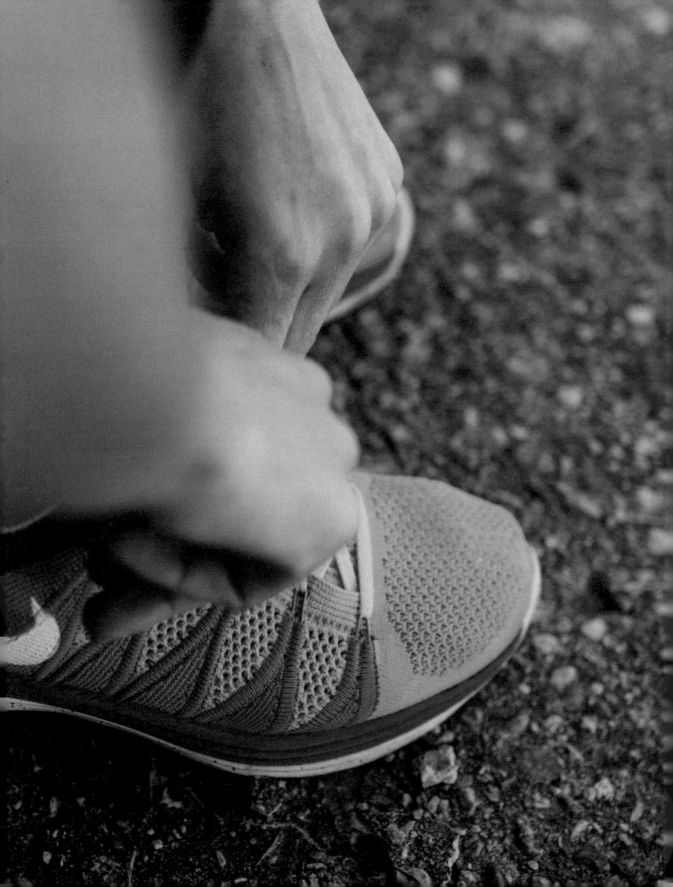

WORKOUTS

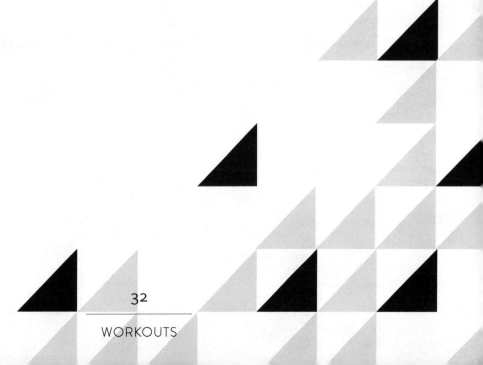

FULL BODY BLASTER

This is a full body strength routine. Do this routine 2-3 times a week or add it to an already established routine and insert it one day to change things up! Grab 2 sets of weights, one lighter and one heavier, (if you only have 1 set, that's ok!) and grab a timer. (Use a kitchen timer or one on your phone! I love the gymboss app!) Be sure to check out the "bonus" section in the welcome for the link to watch a video of how each of these exercises should be done! You can do this workout in 1 of 2 ways:

1 | Do the exercises in the first circuit, 12-15 reps and repeat the circuit again, then move onto the second circuit, repeating again. If you feel up for it, give it one more go, one time through with each circuit!

2 | Set a timer and do each exercise for 1 minute! Give yourself a quick break before moving onto the next one. Rest as you need during that minute. If you are able to move through the exercises without resting during that minute, you need to go harder or heavier! Each circuit will be done twice!

5 MINUTE WARM-UP OF YOUR CHOICE!

CIRCUIT 1	CIRCUIT 2
RENEGADE ROW WITH FROG HOP	THRUSTERS
HINGE SQUAT	SINGLE LEG LUNGE LEAN WITH PRESS (SWITCH LEGS HALFWAY THROUGH)
SURRENDER	PLIE WITH CURL
ELEVATED LUNGE TWIST (SWITCH LEGS HALFWAY THROUGH)	EXTEND & PRESS WITH BALANCE (SWITCH LEGS HALFWAY THROUGH)
30 SECONDS BURPEES	30 SECONDS PLANK JACKS

CARDIO + CORE

This is a cardio and core routine. Do this routine on the days you aren't doing the full body blaster! Aim for 2 days a week! Grab a timer (use the one on your phone!) and get some space around you. Do this circuit 2 - 3 times through! 1 minute of these activities is NO JOKE, but that's how I want it! Rest as you need during the minute and then get back to it. Go hard! Be sure to check out the "bonus" section in the welcome for the link to watch a video of how each of these exercises should be done!

1 4 CORNER HOPS (1 MINUTE)

REST (15 SECONDS)

SPIDER CRAWL (45 SECONDS)

3 PLANK JACKS (1 MINUTE)

REST (15 SECONDS)

BREAST STROKE (45 SECONDS)

2 JUMP KICK (1 MINUTE; SWITCH LEGS AT 30 SECONDS)

REST (15 SECONDS)

ROW YOUR BOAT (45 SECONDS)

4 STAR JUMPS (1 MINUTE)

REST (15 SECONDS)

GRAB THE ROPE (45 SECONDS)

5 BURPEES (1 MINUTE)

REST (15 SECONDS)

PENGUIN TAPS (45 SECONDS: SWITCH SIDES AT 20 SECONDS)

RENEGADE ROW WITH FROG HOP

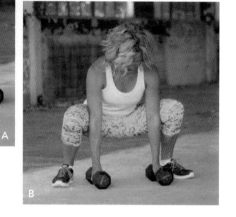

Take your heavy weights and go to all 4's on the ground. Row your right arm up and down and then your left arm up and down as you keep your hips square with the ground. Jump both legs into a frog hop. (Feet should come close to your hands and your hips are sinking down) And then shoot them back out into a plank. Row again and repeat.

HINGE SQUAT

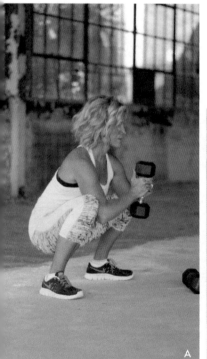
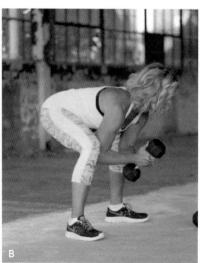

Take 1 heavy weight and squat down to the floor with your legs wide. Place your elbows into your knees and drop your hips. Lift up, leading with your tailbone and come up to where your back is flat and drop back down. Really "sink" in your hips.

SURRENDER

Start holding your lighter weights, one in each hand with your arms above your head. Kneel down with your right leg and then bring your left leg down beside it. Take your right leg and stand up (left leg following) and that's one rep. Halfway through, switch the leg that starts! (left leg steps up first, then right leg follows) To modify: don't hold weights.

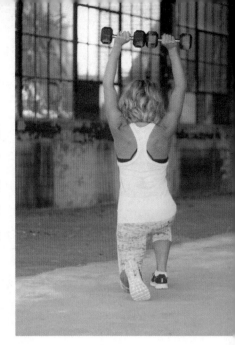

ELEVATED LUNGE TWIST

Place one leg on a bench, chair, or step behind you. (Not recommended to do it as I have in the picture!) Place your hands behind your head and drop down into a lunge. Twist from the waist towards the leg on the ground and come back to starting position. Switch legs halfway through.

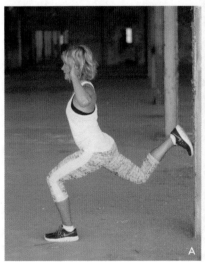

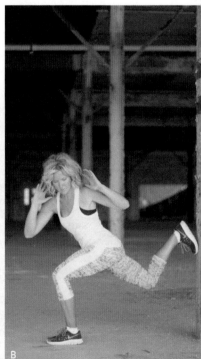

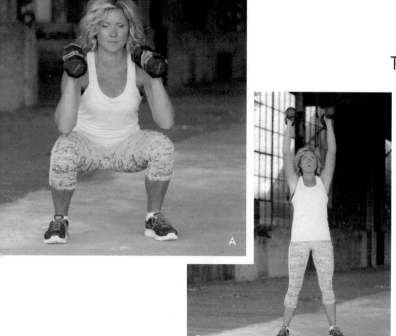

THRUSTERS

Start with a heavy weight in each hand, wrists facing each other. Drop down into a deep squat (legs about hip-width apart) and as you stand, press the weights into the air in one movement.

SINGLE LEG LUNGE LEAN WITH PRESS

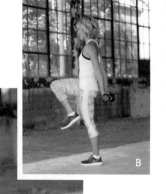

Start in a single-leg lunge with a weight in each hand. Lean from the waist and let your chest hit the top of the leg, then come back up as you bring the back leg up, bent in front of you and press the arms back. Repeat. Switch legs halfway through.

PLIE WITH CURL

Take your heavy weights and hold one in each hand. Place your legs in a "plie" position (widen your legs and turn your feet out) and squat down as you curl your arms up. As you squat down and up, I want you to imagine that I'm "zipping up" the inner and outer thighs. Keep your chest tall. (Don't buckle in the waist!) Keep your elbows pinned at your hips, wrists facing up!

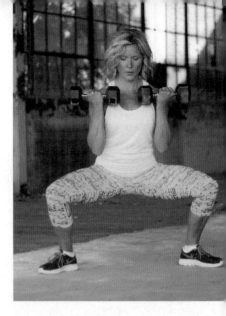

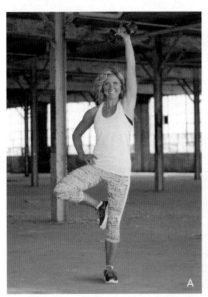

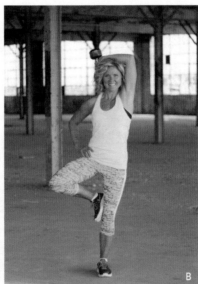

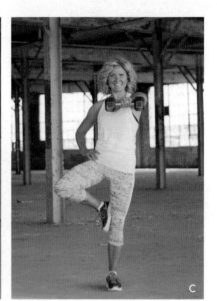

EXTEND & PRESS WITH BALANCE

Take one light weight and hold it above your head. Take the opposite leg and place it at your inner thigh/knee. (To modify, place at floor or ankle) Bend your arm at the elbow and extend up and repeat. Slowly drop the weight in front of you and raise and drop and raise again as you bring it to starting position. Repeat. Switch legs/arms halfway through.

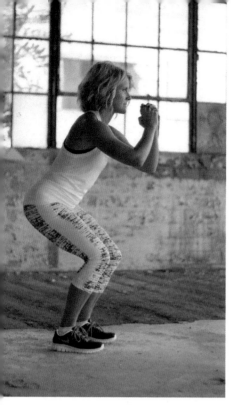

4 CORNER HOPS

Imagine you have a square in front of you. Stand on the "bottom left corner" and jump to the top left corner. Then jump to the top right corner, and then jump to the bottom right corner and then back to the beginning. Reverse the hop around the square. As you jump, land gently. Swing those arms for more power! The bigger the square, the tougher this will be so to modify, keep your square small.

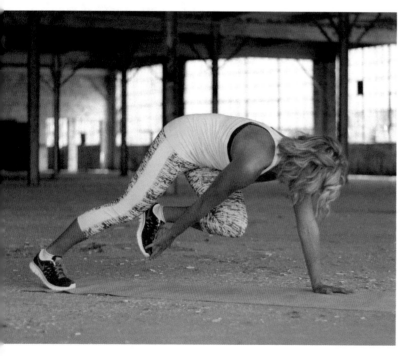

SPIDER CRAWL

Get on all 4's on a mat. Take your right hand as you lift your left foot towards the center and touch it. Return to starting position. Repeat on the other side. To modify, touch elbow to knee!

JUMP KICK

Start standing. Reach your right leg back, step center and then kick with your left leg. To make it harder, add a jump kick!

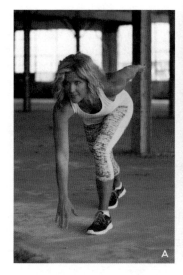
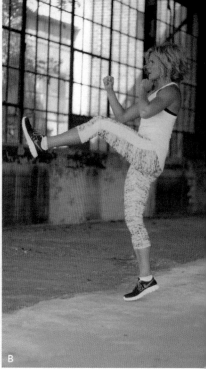

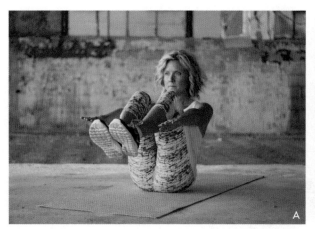
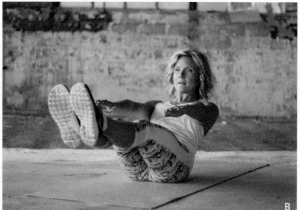

ROW YOUR BOAT

Sit on the floor and lift your legs in the air, knees bent. Reach arms out to the side and then lean back as you extend your legs out, balancing on your sitz bones. Bring your knees back in toward your chest and repeat!

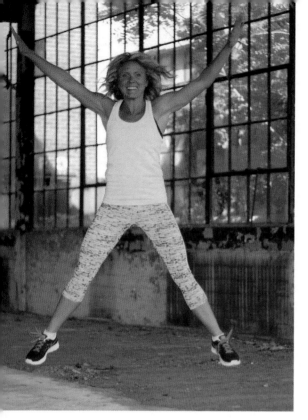

STAR JUMPS

Start with hands crossed in front of your ankles or shins. Jump high and wide as you extend your arms and legs like a big star!

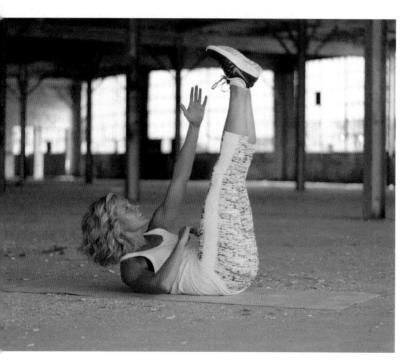

GRAB THE ROPE

Lay on your back. Imagine there is a rope hanging from the ceiling and reach for it, grabbing right and left. To make it harder, lift your shoulder blades off the mat and to make it easier, lean back on the mat!

BURPEES

Start in a standing position. Drop straight down with hands to the floor and then kick the legs back into a plank. Jump your legs back to your hands and stand up. To make it harder, jump up. To make it easier step one leg back and then the other.

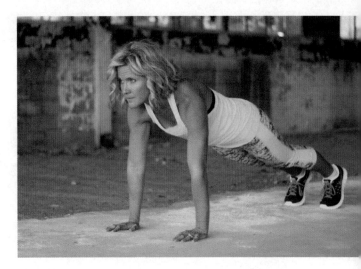

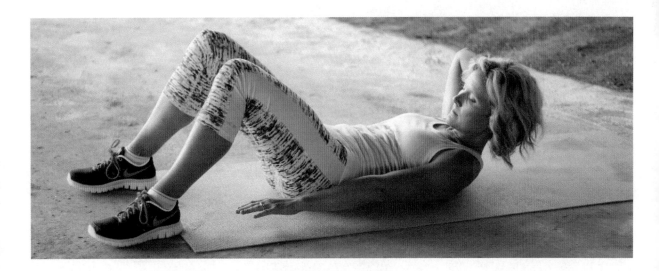

PENGUIN TAPS

Lay on your back with your legs bent. Place one hand behind your head and take the other hand and reach it towards your ankles. Imagine that I have a knob on the top of your chest and I'm turning you. It is a shift to the side. Do not raise up on the other shoulder. If it doesn't hurt your neck, you can remove your hands fro your neck and keep both hands at the ankles and alternate the tap!

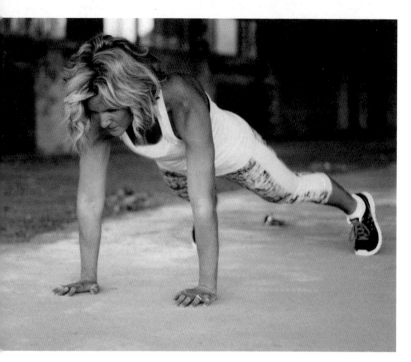

PLANK JACKS

Go onto all 4's on the ground. Keep your hands steady and move your feet out and in as if you are doing a jumping jack.

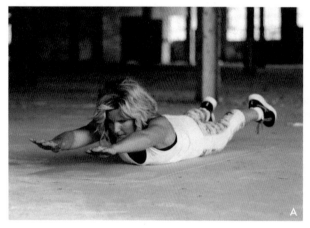

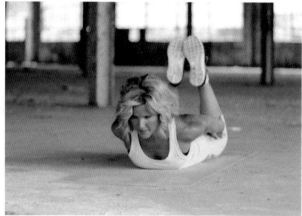

BREAST STROKE

Go onto your belly on the mat and extend your arms in front of you, legs behind you. Reach your arms out and around as if you are going to grab your ankles as you bend your legs towards your bottom. Extend your arms and legs back to starting position. To make this harder, lift the chest a little higher and to make it easier, keep the chest lower to the mat.

living + active

HEBREWS 4:12

word-fed

NOT

FOOD LED

spirit-led

NOT

FLESH FED

TIED TOGETHER (Ecclesiastes 4:12, Proverbs 27:17)

DEDICATED DAILY (Matthew 6:34, Lamentations 3:22-23)

CRAVING CONQUERERS (1 John 2:16, Psalm 107:9)

HEART HEALTHY (Proverbs 4:23, Psalm 73:26)

MARATHON MINDED (1 Thessalonians 5:23, Galatians 6:9)

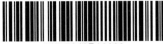

Made in the USA
Lexington, KY
09 October 2015